LIFESPAN DIET COOKBOOK

Unlocking the Culinary Fountain of Youth – Decoding the Secrets of Aging and Empowering You to Defy the Clock

Lori J. Garcia

Table of Contents

CHAPTER 3: WHOLESOME LUNCHES FOR LONGEVITY

INTRODUCTION

Welcome to the Lifespan Diet Cookbook

Where the culinary arts meet the science of aging in a groundbreaking exploration of longevity. In a world saturated with diets promising quick fixes, this cookbook stands apart, offering more than just recipes; it unveils the keys to understanding the intricacies of aging and empowers you to take control of your own biological clock.

Have you ever wondered why some cultures seem to age gracefully, maintaining vitality well into their later years? The Lifespan Diet Cookbook holds the answers, blending the wisdom of age-old culinary traditions with cutting-edge scientific research.

Embark on a journey beyond the ordinary, as we unravel the mysteries of aging and reveal how the food on your plate can be a powerful tool in defying the passage of time. This is not just a cookbook; it's a guide to a lifestyle that challenges the status quo, proving that aging is not an inevitable decline but a malleable aspect of our existence.

Join us as we navigate the intersection of delectable cuisine and the science of longevity. Each recipe is a step towards a healthier, more vibrant life, backed by the latest research on nutrition, cellular health, and the secrets of cultures renowned for their enduring well-being.

The Lifespan Diet Cookbook transcends the boundaries of traditional diet guides. It's a holistic approach that considers not only what you eat but how it impacts your body at the cellular level. Say goodbye to restrictive diets and welcome a culinary adventure that nourishes not just your taste buds but your entire being.

This isn't just about adding years to your life; it's about adding life to your years. The Lifespan Diet Cookbook is your companion on the journey to a future where aging is a choice, not a mandate. Are you ready to embrace a life filled with vitality, flavor, and the delightful anticipation of many more healthy, happy years? Let's begin.

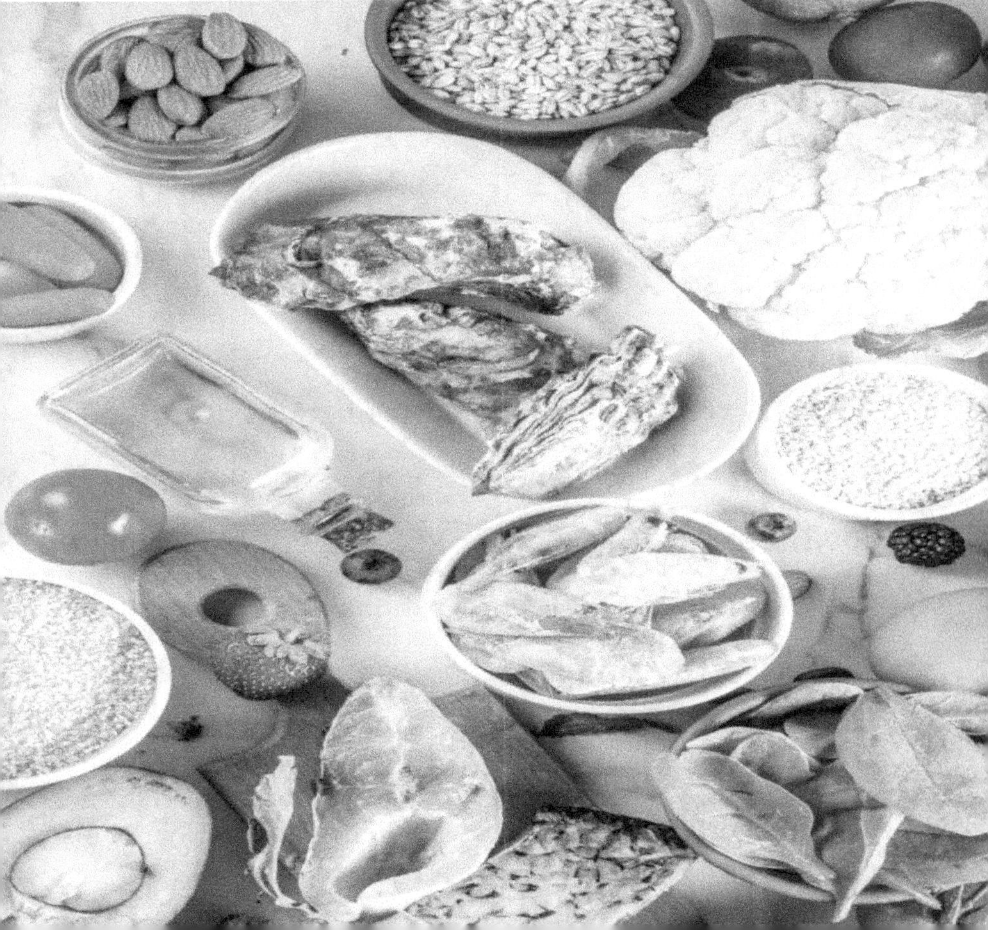

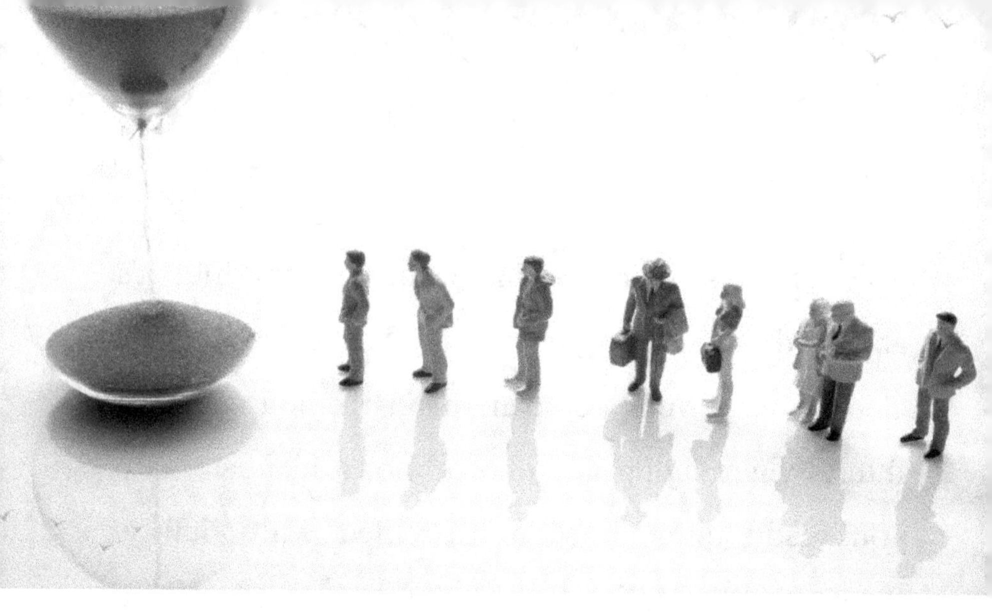

CHAPTER 1: THE CULINARY KEY TO LONGEVITY

The Role of Nutrition in Lifespan Extension

In the quest for a longer and healthier life, the role of nutrition emerges as a pivotal factor, and it is this very premise that forms the essence of the Lifespan Diet. Beyond the conventional view of food merely as sustenance, this dietary philosophy delves into the intricate relationship between the nutrients we consume and the extension of our lifespan.

At its core, the Lifespan Diet advocates for a mindful and intentional approach to nutrition, considering the quality of food over mere caloric intake. Nutrient density takes center stage, emphasizing the consumption of foods rich in vitamins, minerals, and antioxidants. These components act as powerful agents in combating cellular damage, a key contributor to the aging process.

The Lifespan Diet Pyramid serves as a guiding framework, illustrating the optimal proportions of various food groups for a balanced and longevity-promoting diet. It goes beyond the one-size-fits-all mentality of traditional dietary guidelines, recognizing the individualized nature of nutritional needs for a diverse population.

Superfoods become the unsung heroes in this narrative, celebrated for their exceptional nutrient profiles and potential to support cellular health. Antioxidants, in particular, play a crucial role in neutralizing free radicals, thereby reducing oxidative stress on cells and tissues.

However, the Lifespan Diet is not a mere catalog of foods; it's a comprehensive lifestyle approach. Balancing macronutrients, strategically timing meals, and adopting mindful eating practices are all integral components. This dietary philosophy recognizes the importance of hydration, the impact of culinary techniques on nutrient retention, and the profound connection between what we eat and how we age.

Building a Foundation of Sustainable Eating Habits

Building a foundation of sustainable eating habits is the cornerstone of the Lifespan Diet, transcending the transient allure of fad diets and quick fixes. At its essence, sustainability in this context encompasses not only the environmental impact of our food choices but also the long-term viability of our dietary patterns in promoting overall health and longevity.

In the world of the Lifespan Diet, sustainability begins with an awareness of the sources and production methods of the foods we consume. Embracing locally sourced, seasonal, and organic options becomes a conscious choice, contributing to environmental stewardship while prioritizing the nutritional integrity of our meals.

The foundation of sustainable eating extends beyond the environmental realm to the very core of our individual well-being. The Lifespan Diet encourages a balanced and varied intake of whole foods, emphasizing the consumption of fruits, vegetables, whole grains, lean proteins, and healthy fats. This diverse palette not only provides a spectrum of essential nutrients but also supports the body's intricate systems for optimal function.

One of the key tenets of sustainability within the Lifespan Diet is the notion of moderation and portion control. Rather than subscribing to restrictive eating practices, the emphasis is on mindful consumption. Understanding hunger cues and cultivating an attuned relationship with food are integral components of sustainable eating habits, fostering a balanced approach that can be maintained over the long term.

Moreover, the Lifespan Diet acknowledges the social and cultural aspects of eating, promoting the enjoyment of meals as a communal and pleasurable experience. This recognition of food as more than just fuel aligns with the sustainable nature of a dietary approach that can seamlessly integrate into diverse lifestyles.

Cellular Health and Its Impact on Longevity

In the intricate dance of life, cellular health emerges as a fundamental determinant of longevity, and the Lifespan Diet places this concept at the forefront of its philosophy. At its essence, the lifespan of an organism is intricately woven into the health of its individual cells. The Lifespan Diet delves into the cellular landscape, recognizing that the cumulative well-being of these microscopic powerhouses dictates the overall trajectory of an individual's life span.

Understanding cellular health within the context of the Lifespan Diet involves appreciating the role of genetics, lifestyle, and environmental factors in influencing the intricate balance of our cells. The diet acknowledges that our cells are constantly engaged in a delicate interplay, responding to the nutrients we consume, the stresses we experience, and the overall quality of our lifestyle choices.

At the heart of this dietary philosophy is the recognition that cellular damage, particularly oxidative stress, plays a pivotal role in the aging process. Free radicals, generated through various metabolic processes and environmental exposures, can wreak havoc on cellular structures. The Lifespan Diet counteracts this by promoting an antioxidant-rich nutritional profile, derived from foods like berries, leafy greens, and other nutrient-dense options. Antioxidants act as cellular defenders, neutralizing free radicals and mitigating the impact of oxidative stress.

The Lifespan Diet further underscores the importance of maintaining cellular integrity through proper hydration, strategic meal timing, and the incorporation of essential nutrients. Balanced macronutrients, including healthy fats, proteins, and carbohydrates, contribute to the resilience and functionality of cells, ensuring they operate optimally.

Balancing Macronutrients for Optimal Health

In the intricate tapestry of the Lifespan Diet, the concept of balancing macronutrients emerges as a central pillar, orchestrating a symphony of health within the body. Macronutrients – proteins, fats, and carbohydrates – are the essential building blocks that fuel our physiological processes and sustain life. The Lifespan Diet intricately examines the delicate equilibrium of these macronutrients, recognizing that their balanced interplay is crucial for optimal health and longevity.

Proteins, the body's structural backbone, play a pivotal role in cellular repair, immune function, and the synthesis of essential molecules. The Lifespan Diet advocates for a balanced intake of high-quality proteins, sourced from lean meats, legumes, and plant-based alternatives, fostering cellular resilience and fortitude.

Healthy fats, another cornerstone of the Lifespan Diet, are dispelling the myth that all fats are detrimental. Embracing sources like avocados, nuts, seeds, and fatty fish, the diet acknowledges the role of fats in cellular membrane integrity, hormone production, and the absorption of fat-soluble vitamins. It encourages a mindful incorporation of these essential fats for a well-rounded and nourishing dietary profile.

Carbohydrates, often at the heart of dietary debates, are approached with nuance in the Lifespan Diet.

Emphasizing complex carbohydrates derived from whole grains, fruits, and vegetables, the diet champions sustained energy release and optimal blood sugar control. It advocates steering away from refined sugars and processed carbs, recognizing the impact of such choices on inflammation and metabolic health.

By navigating the delicate balance of these macronutrients, the Lifespan Diet aims to optimize the body's internal environment. It acknowledges that the unique composition of each individual requires personalized adjustments, and its guidelines serve as a flexible framework adaptable to diverse lifestyles.

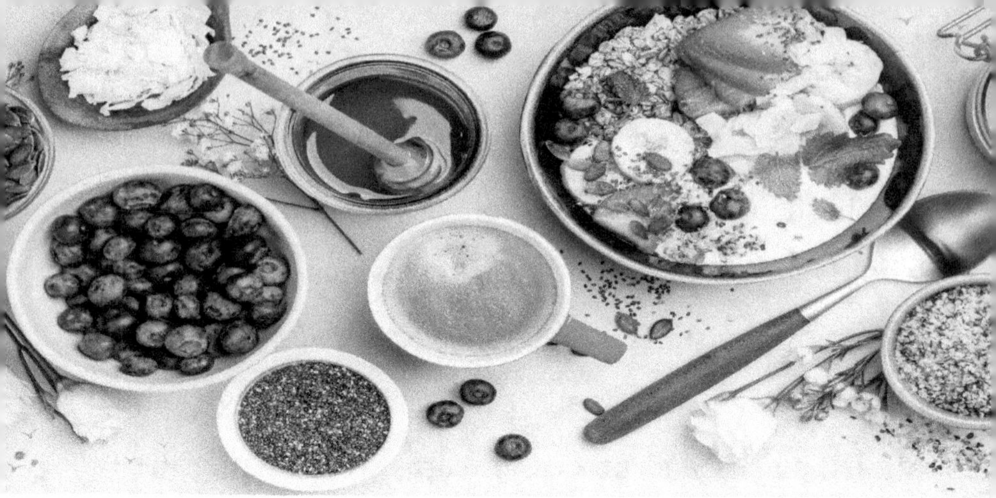

CHAPTER 2: TRANSFORMATIVE BREAKFASTS

Mediterranean Morning Delight:

Ingredients:

- 3 eggs
- 1 medium tomato, diced
- 1/4 cup Kalamata olives, sliced
- 2 tbsp feta cheese, crumbled
- 1 tsp oregano
- Salt and pepper to taste
- 2 slices whole-grain bread, toasted

1. In a bowl, beat the eggs and season with salt and pepper.
2. In a non-stick pan, scramble the eggs until almost set.
3. Add diced tomatoes, olives, and crumbled feta. Continue cooking until eggs are fully set.
4. Sprinkle with oregano and serve over toasted whole-grain bread.

Prep Time: *15 minutes*

✓ *Rich in protein for sustained energy.*
✓ *Provides essential vitamins and minerals from tomatoes and olives.*
✓ *Whole-grain bread offers fiber for digestive health.*

Sunrise Quinoa Bowl:

Ingredients:

- 1 cup quinoa
- 2 cups almond milk
- 1 cup mixed berries (strawberries, blueberries, raspberries)
- 1/4 cup chopped nuts (almonds, walnuts)
- Honey for drizzling

Instructions:

1. Rinse quinoa and cook it in almond milk according to package instructions.
2. Once cooked, divide quinoa into bowls.
3. Top with mixed berries, chopped nuts, and a drizzle of honey.

Prep Time: *20 minutes*

- ✓ *Quinoa provides a complete protein source.*
- ✓ *Almond milk adds a dose of vitamin E and healthy fats.*
- ✓ *Berries offer antioxidants for cellular health.*

Veggie-Packed Shakshuka:

Ingredients:

- 4 eggs
- 1 can (14 oz) crushed tomatoes
- 1 red bell pepper, diced
- 1 onion, finely chopped
- 2 cloves garlic, minced
- 1 tsp cumin
- 1 tsp paprika
- Salt and pepper to taste
- Fresh parsley for garnish

Instructions:

1. In a skillet, sauté onions and bell pepper until softened. Add garlic and spices, cook for another minute.
2. Pour in crushed tomatoes and simmer for 10 minutes.

3. Make wells in the sauce and crack eggs into them. Cover and cook until eggs are done to your liking.

4. Garnish with fresh parsley and serve.

Prep Time: *25 minutes*

✓ *High in lycopene from tomatoes, promoting heart health.*

✓ *Eggs provide complete protein.*

✓ *Bell peppers are rich in vitamin C for immune support.*

Mango & Avocado Smoothie Bowl:

Ingredients:

- 1 ripe mango, peeled and diced
- 1 ripe avocado, peeled and pitted
- Handful of spinach
- 1/2 cup Greek yogurt
- 1/2 cup almond milk
- 1 tbsp chia seeds

- Mixed berries for topping

Instructions:

1. Blend mango, avocado, spinach, Greek yogurt, and almond milk until smooth.
2. Pour into a bowl, top with chia seeds and mixed berries.

Prep Time: *10 minutes*

✓ *Avocado and chia seeds provide healthy fats for satiety.*

✓ *Spinach offers iron and other essential nutrients.*

✓ *Greek yogurt adds probiotics for gut health.*

Plant-Powered Overnight Oats:

Ingredients:

- 1 cup rolled oats
- 1 cup almond milk
- 1 banana, sliced
- 2 tbsp chia seeds

- 1 tbsp almond butter

Instructions:

1. In a jar, combine rolled oats and almond milk. Stir in sliced banana and chia seeds.
2. Refrigerate overnight.
3. Before serving, top with a dollop of almond butter.

Prep Time: *5 minutes (plus overnight refrigeration)*

- ✓ *Oats offer soluble fiber for heart health.*
- ✓ *Chia seeds provide omega-3 fatty acids.*
- ✓ *Almond butter adds protein and healthy fats.*

Anti-Inflammatory Turmeric Scramble:

Ingredients:

- ✓ 1 block tofu, crumbled
- 1 tsp turmeric
- 1/2 tsp black pepper
- 1 cup spinach, chopped

- Salt to taste
- Quinoa or whole-grain toast for serving

1. In a skillet, sauté crumbled tofu with turmeric and black pepper until golden.
2. Add chopped spinach and cook until wilted.
3. Season with salt and serve over quinoa or whole-grain toast.

Prep Time: 15 minutes

✓ *Turmeric has anti-inflammatory properties.*
✓ *Tofu provides a plant-based protein source.*
✓ *Spinach is rich in iron and vitamins.*

Berry-licious Acai Bowl:

Ingredients:

- 1 packet frozen acai puree
- 1/2 cup mixed berries
- 1/2 cup almond milk

- Granola, sliced kiwi, and agave syrup for topping

Instructions:

1. Blend acai puree, mixed berries, and almond milk until smooth.
2. Pour into a bowl, top with granola, sliced kiwi, and a drizzle of agave syrup.

Prep Time: *10 minutes*

✓ *Acai is rich in antioxidants.*

✓ *Mixed berries provide vitamins and fiber.*

✓ *Almond milk offers a dairy-free alternative.*

Chia Seed Pudding Parfait:

Ingredients:

- 1/4 cup chia seeds
- 1 cup coconut yogurt
- Mixed berries

- Crushed almonds

Instructions:

1. Mix chia seeds with coconut yogurt and refrigerate for a few hours or overnight.
2. In a glass, layer chia pudding with mixed berries and crushed almonds.

Prep Time: *5 minutes (plus chilling time)*

- ✓ *Chia seeds provide omega-3 fatty acids and fiber.*
- ✓ *Coconut yogurt offers a dairy-free probiotic option.*
- ✓ *Berries contribute antioxidants for cellular health.*

Tomato Basil Frittata:

Ingredients:

- 6 eggs
- 1 cup cherry tomatoes, halved
- 1/4 cup fresh basil, chopped

- 1/2 cup goat cheese, crumbled
- Salt and pepper to taste

Instructions:

1. Preheat oven to 350°F (175°C).
2. Whisk eggs and season with salt and pepper.
3. Pour into a greased baking dish, add tomatoes, basil, and goat cheese.
4. Bake for 20-25 minutes or until set.

Prep Time: *15 minutes*

- ✓ *Eggs provide a high-quality protein source.*
- ✓ *Tomatoes and basil offer vitamins and antioxidants.*
- ✓ *Goat cheese adds a creamy texture and flavor.*

Green Goddess Smoothie:

Ingredients:

- ✓ Handful of spinach
- ✓ Handful of kale

- ✓ 1 cup pineapple chunks
- ✓ 1 banana
- ✓ 1/2 cup coconut water
- ✓ Mint leaves for garnish

Instructions:

1. Blend spinach, kale, pineapple, banana, and coconut water until smooth.
2. Pour into a glass, garnish with mint leaves.

Prep Time: *10 minutes*

- ✓ *Spinach and kale are rich in vitamins and minerals.*
- ✓ *Pineapple adds natural sweetness and vitamin C.*
- ✓ *Coconut water provides hydration and electrolytes.*

Protein-Packed Lentil Pancakes:

Ingredients:

- 1 cup lentil flour

- 1/2 cup water
- 1 tsp baking powder
- 1 tbsp maple syrup
- Greek yogurt, berries, and maple syrup for topping

Instructions:

1. Mix lentil flour, water, baking powder, and maple syrup until well combined.
2. Cook pancakes on a griddle until golden.
3. Top with Greek yogurt, berries, and a drizzle of maple syrup.

Prep Time: *15 minutes*

✓ *Lentil flour provides a protein and fiber boost.*
✓ *Greek yogurt adds probiotics for gut health.*
✓ *Berries offer antioxidants and natural sweetness.*

Olive & Herb Omelette:

Ingredients:

- 4 eggs
- 1/4 cup Kalamata olives, sliced
- 1/2 cup cherry tomatoes, halved
- Fresh herbs (such as parsley or basil), chopped
- Salt and pepper to taste

Instructions:

1. Whisk eggs and season with salt and pepper.
2. Pour into a heated, greased pan.
3. Add olives, cherry tomatoes, and fresh herbs.
4. Cook until the edges set, then fold in half.

Prep Time: *10 minutes*

- ✓ *Olives provide healthy monounsaturated fats.*
- ✓ *Tomatoes and herbs offer vitamins and antioxidants.*
- ✓ *Eggs contribute high-quality protein.*

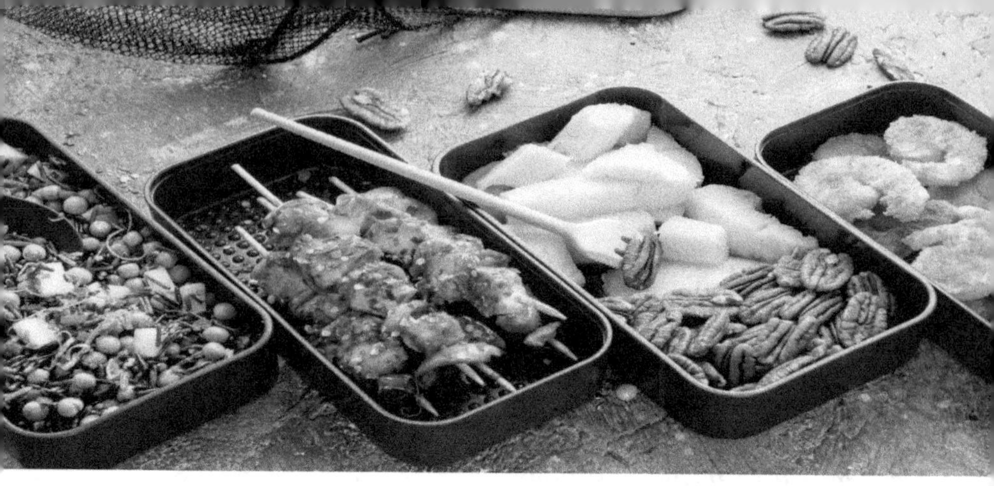

CHAPTER 3: WHOLESOME LUNCHES FOR LONGEVITY

Mediterranean Quinoa Salad:

Ingredients:

- 1 cup cooked quinoa
- Cherry tomatoes, cucumber, red onion (diced)
- Kalamata olives, feta cheese
- Fresh parsley, olive oil, lemon juice
- Salt and pepper to taste

Instructions:

1. Mix quinoa with chopped vegetables, olives, and feta.

2. Drizzle with olive oil, lemon juice, and season.

3. Toss well and refrigerate before serving.

Prep Time: 15 minutes

✓ *Quinoa provides complete protein.*

✓ *Vegetables offer fiber and antioxidants.*

✓ *Olive oil supports heart health.*

Chickpea and Spinach Stew:

Ingredients:

- 1 can chickpeas, drained
- Spinach, tomatoes, carrots (chopped)
- Garlic, cumin, paprika, vegetable broth
- Salt and pepper to taste

Instructions:

1. Sauté garlic, add vegetables, and spices.

2. Pour in vegetable broth, add chickpeas, and simmer.

3. Season to taste and serve warm.

Prep Time: *20 minutes*

✓ *Chickpeas provide protein and fiber.*

✓ *Spinach offers vitamins and iron.*

✓ *Anti-inflammatory spices enhance health.*

Mushroom and Lentil Stuffed Peppers:

Ingredients:

- Bell peppers (halved)
- Lentils, mushrooms, onions (cooked)
- Tomato sauce, Italian herbs
- Mozzarella cheese (optional)

Instructions:

1. Mix lentils, mushrooms, onions, and herbs.
2. Stuff peppers, top with tomato sauce, and bake.
3. Add mozzarella in the last 5 minutes if desired.

Prep Time: *25 minutes*

✓ *Lentils offer protein and fiber.*

✓ *Mushrooms provide antioxidants.*

✓ *Bell peppers are rich in vitamin C.*

Plant-Based Buddha Bowl:

Ingredients:

- Quinoa or brown rice
- Roasted sweet potatoes, broccoli, and chickpeas
- Avocado slices, hummus
- Tahini dressing

Instructions:

1. Arrange quinoa, roasted veggies, and chickpeas.
2. Add avocado, dollops of hummus, and drizzle with tahini.

Prep Time: *30 minutes*

✓ *Balanced plant-based proteins.*

✓ *Sweet potatoes offer vitamins and fiber.*

✓ *Healthy fats from avocado and tahini.*

Lemon Garlic Salmon with Asparagus:

Ingredients:

- Salmon fillets
- Asparagus spears
- Garlic, lemon juice, olive oil
- Fresh dill, salt, and pepper

Instructions:

1. Season salmon with garlic, lemon, and dill.
2. Roast salmon and asparagus in olive oil.
3. Serve with a squeeze of fresh lemon.

Prep Time: *20 minutes*

- ✓ *Salmon provides omega-3 fatty acids.*
- ✓ *Asparagus is rich in vitamins and fiber.*
- ✓ *Garlic and lemon add flavor and antioxidants.*

Quinoa and Black Bean Stuffed Zucchini:

Ingredients:

- Zucchini (halved and scooped)
- Quinoa, black beans, corn
- Onion, cumin, chili powder
- Salsa, cilantro, lime wedges

Instructions:

1. Sauté onion, add quinoa, beans, and spices.
2. Stuff zucchini, bake until tender.
3. Top with salsa, cilantro, and a squeeze of lime.

Prep Time: *25 minutes*

- ✓ *Quinoa and black beans offer protein.*
- ✓ *Zucchini provides vitamins and fiber.*
- ✓ *Fresh salsa adds antioxidants.*

Turmeric Lentil Soup:

Ingredients:

- Red lentils, carrots, celery, onion
- Garlic, turmeric, cumin, coriander
- Vegetable broth, coconut milk

- Fresh cilantro, lime wedges

1. Sauté garlic, add lentils, vegetables, and spices.
2. Pour in vegetable broth, simmer until lentils are cooked.
3. Stir in coconut milk, garnish with cilantro and lime.

Prep Time: *30 minutes*

✓ *Lentils offer protein and iron.*
✓ *Turmeric has anti-inflammatory properties.*
✓ *Vegetables add vitamins and fiber.*

Avocado and Chickpea Wrap:

Ingredients:

- Whole-grain wrap
- Mashed avocado, chickpeas (mashed)
- Cherry tomatoes, cucumber, lettuce
- Hummus, lemon juice, salt, and pepper

Instructions:

1. Spread mashed avocado and chickpeas on the wrap.
2. Add sliced tomatoes, cucumber, and lettuce.
3. Drizzle with hummus, lemon juice, and season.

Prep Time: *15 minutes*

✓ *Avocado provides healthy fats.*

✓ *Chickpeas offer protein and fiber.*

✓ *Whole-grain wrap adds complex carbs.*

Eggplant and Tomato Ratatouille:

Ingredients:

- Eggplant, zucchini, bell peppers (sliced)
- Onion, garlic, tomatoes (chopped)
- Fresh thyme, rosemary
- Olive oil, salt, and pepper

Instructions:

1. Sauté onion and garlic, add sliced vegetables.

2. Stir in tomatoes, thyme, and rosemary.

3. Roast until vegetables are tender.

Prep Time: *20 minutes*

✓ *Eggplant and zucchini offer fiber.*

✓ *Tomatoes provide antioxidants.*

✓ *Fresh herbs add flavor and nutrients.*

Quinoa and Edamame Salad:

Ingredients:

- Cooked quinoa
- Edamame, cucumber, radishes (sliced)
- Sesame oil, soy sauce, rice vinegar
- Sesame seeds, green onions

Instructions:

1. Mix quinoa with edamame, cucumber, and radishes.

2. Whisk together sesame oil, soy sauce, and rice vinegar.

3. Drizzle dressing over the salad, top with sesame seeds and green onions.

Prep Time: *15 minutes*

✓ *Quinoa offers complete protein.*

✓ *Edamame is rich in plant-based protein.*

✓ *Sesame seeds provide healthy fats.*

Spinach and Lentil Stuffed Bell Peppers:

Ingredients:

- Bell peppers (halved)
- Cooked lentils, spinach, tomatoes (chopped)
- Onion, garlic, Italian herbs
- Feta cheese (optional)

Instructions:

1. Sauté onion and garlic, add lentils, spinach, and tomatoes.

2. Stuff peppers, sprinkle with Italian herbs, and
    bake.

3. Add feta in the last 5 minutes if desired.

Prep Time: *25 minutes*

✓ *Lentils provide protein and fiber.*

✓ *Spinach offers vitamins and iron.*

✓ *Bell peppers are rich in vitamin C.*

Cauliflower and Chickpea Curry:

Ingredients:

- Cauliflower florets, chickpeas
- Onion, garlic, ginger (minced)
- Curry powder, turmeric, cumin
- Coconut milk, tomatoes (diced)
- Fresh cilantro, lime wedges

Instructions:

1. Sauté onion, garlic, and ginger. Add cauliflower
    and chickpeas.

2. Stir in curry powder, turmeric, and cumin.

3. Pour in coconut milk, add diced tomatoes, and simmer.

4. Garnish with cilantro and serve with lime wedges.

Prep Time: *30 minutes*

✓ *Chickpeas provide protein and fiber.*

✓ *Cauliflower offers vitamins and antioxidants.*

✓ *Turmeric and cumin have anti-inflammatory properties.*

Mediterranean Chickpea Salad:

Ingredients:

- Chickpeas (canned or cooked)
- Cherry tomatoes, cucumber, red onion (diced)
- Feta cheese, Kalamata olives
- Fresh parsley, olive oil, lemon juice
- Salt and pepper to taste

1. Mix chickpeas with chopped vegetables, olives, and feta.
2. Drizzle with olive oil, lemon juice, and season.
3. Toss well and refrigerate before serving.

Prep Time: *15 minutes*

✓ *Chickpeas provide protein and fiber.*

✓ *Vegetables offer vitamins and antioxidants.*

✓ *Olive oil supports heart health.*

Sweet Potato and Black Bean Burrito Bowl:

Ingredients:

- Roasted sweet potatoes
- Black beans (canned or cooked)
- Brown rice, corn, avocado
- Salsa, lime wedges, cilantro

Instructions:

1. Arrange brown rice, roasted sweet potatoes, and black beans.

2. Add corn, avocado slices, and drizzle with salsa.

3. Garnish with lime wedges and fresh cilantro.

Prep Time: 25 minutes

✓ *Sweet potatoes offer vitamins and fiber.*

✓ *Black beans provide protein and fiber.*

✓ *Avocado adds healthy fats.*

Stuffed Portobello Mushrooms:

Ingredients:

- Portobello mushrooms (stem removed)
- Quinoa, spinach, cherry tomatoes (cooked)
- Garlic, balsamic vinegar, olive oil
- Goat cheese, pine nuts (optional)

Instructions:

1. Sauté garlic, add cooked quinoa, spinach, and tomatoes.

2. Spoon the mixture into portobello mushrooms.

3. Drizzle with balsamic vinegar, olive oil, and bake.

4. Top with goat cheese and pine nuts if desired.

Prep Time: *20 minutes*

✓ *Quinoa offers complete protein.*

✓ *Spinach provides vitamins and iron.*

✓ *Portobello mushrooms are rich in antioxidants.*

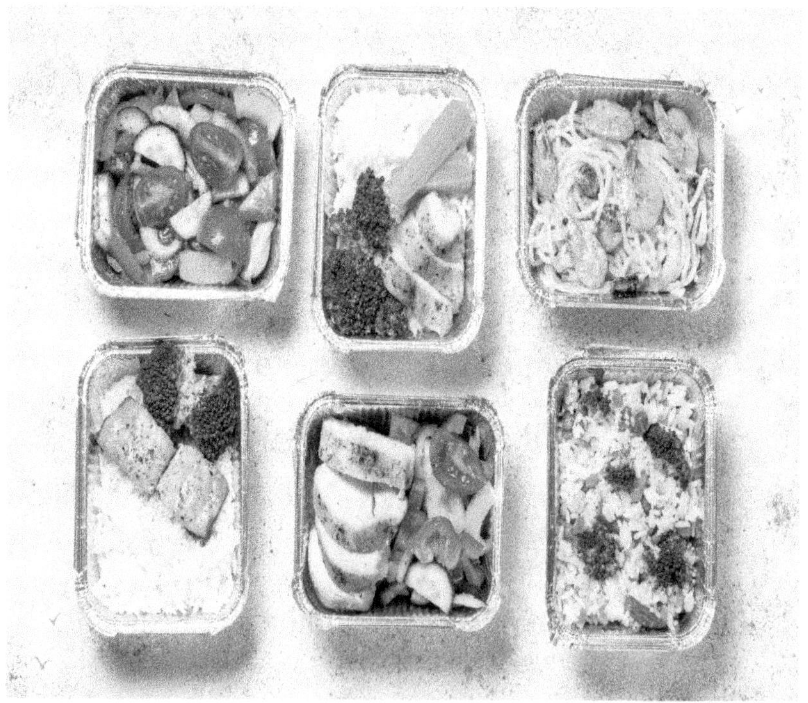

egetables

Legumes

Dairy
products

whole
grains

Seeds

Healthy
fats

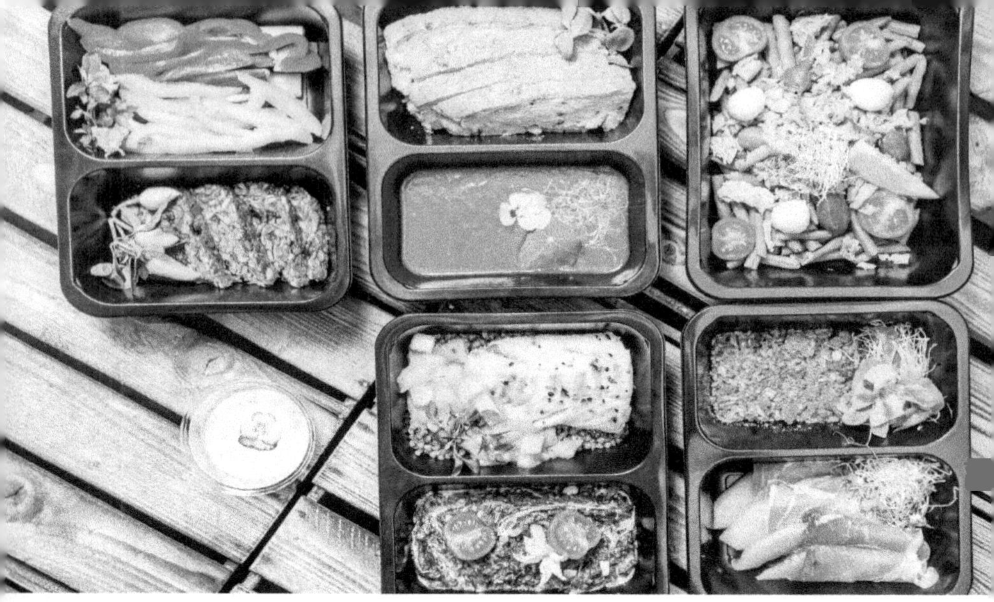

CHAPTER 4: DINNER DELIGHTS FOR A TIMELESS YOU

Mediterranean Baked Cod with Lemon and Herbs:

Ingredients:

- Cod fillets
- Lemon, garlic, fresh dill
- Cherry tomatoes, olives
- Olive oil, salt, and pepper

1. Marinate cod with lemon, garlic, and dill.

2. Place on a bed of cherry tomatoes and olives.

3. Drizzle with olive oil, season, and bake.

Prep Time: *20 minutes*

✓ Cod is rich in omega-3 fatty acids.

✓ Tomatoes and olives offer antioxidants.

✓ Fresh herbs add flavor and nutrients.

Plant-Powered Lentil and Vegetable Stir-Fry:

Ingredients:

● Cooked lentils

● Mixed vegetables (broccoli, bell peppers, carrots)

● Ginger, garlic, soy sauce

● Quinoa or brown rice

Instructions:

1. Sauté ginger and garlic, add vegetables and cooked lentils.

2. Stir in soy sauce, serve over quinoa or brown rice.

Prep Time: *25 minutes*

✓ *Lentils provide protein and fiber.*

✓ *Colorful vegetables offer vitamins.*

✓ *Quinoa or brown rice adds complex carbs.*

Anti-Inflammatory Turmeric Chickpea Curry:

Ingredients:

- Chickpeas, coconut milk
- Onion, garlic, ginger
- Turmeric, cumin, coriander
- Spinach, tomatoes

Instructions:

1. Sauté onion, garlic, and ginger. Add chickpeas, coconut milk, and spices.

2. Stir in spinach and tomatoes, simmer until cooked.

3. Serve over brown rice.

Prep Time: *30 minutes*

✓ *Chickpeas provide protein and fiber.*

✓ *Turmeric has anti-inflammatory properties.*

✓ *Spinach and tomatoes offer vitamins.*

Mushroom and Spinach Stuffed Bell Peppers:

Ingredients:

- Bell peppers (halved)
- Mushrooms, spinach, tomatoes (chopped)
- Onion, garlic, Italian herbs
- Quinoa or couscous

Instructions:

1. Sauté onion and garlic, add mushrooms, spinach, and tomatoes.

2. Mix with cooked quinoa or couscous.

3. Stuff peppers, bake until tender.

Prep Time: *25 minutes*

✓ Mushrooms and spinach provide vitamins.

✓ Bell peppers offer antioxidants.

✓ Quinoa or couscous adds texture and nutrients.

Roasted Eggplant and Chickpea Salad:

Ingredients:

- Eggplant, chickpeas
- Cherry tomatoes, cucumber, red onion
- Feta cheese, olive oil, lemon juice

Instructions:

1. Roast eggplant and chickpeas until golden.

2. Toss with cherry tomatoes, cucumber, and red onion.

3. Drizzle with olive oil and lemon juice, top with feta.

Prep Time: *30 minutes*

✓ *Eggplant and chickpeas provide fiber.*

✓ *Tomatoes and cucumber offer vitamins.*

✓ *Olive oil adds healthy fats.*

Lemon Herb Quinoa with Grilled Vegetables:

Ingredients:

- Quinoa
- Zucchini, bell peppers, asparagus (grilled)
- Lemon, fresh herbs (rosemary, thyme)
- Olive oil, salt, and pepper

Instructions:

1. Cook quinoa according to package instructions.
2. Toss grilled vegetables with quinoa, lemon, and herbs.
3. Drizzle with olive oil, season, and serve.

Prep Time: *35 minutes*

- ✓ *Quinoa provides complete protein.*
- ✓ *Grilled vegetables offer vitamins.*
- ✓ *Fresh herbs add flavor and nutrients.*

Avocado and Chickpea Pasta:

Ingredients:

- Whole-grain or chickpea pasta
- Avocado, cherry tomatoes, arugula
- Garlic, lemon juice, olive oil

Instructions:

1. Cook pasta according to package instructions.
2. Blend avocado, garlic, and lemon juice for the sauce.
3. Toss pasta with the sauce, cherry tomatoes, and arugula.

Prep Time: *20 minutes*

- ✓ *Whole-grain or chickpea pasta offers fiber.*
- ✓ *Avocado provides healthy fats.*

✓ *Tomatoes and arugula offer vitamins.*

Mediterranean Quinoa Stuffed Peppers:

Ingredients:

- Quinoa, black beans
- Cherry tomatoes, Kalamata olives, feta
- Fresh parsley, olive oil, lemon juice

Instructions:

1. Cook quinoa and black beans.
2. Mix with tomatoes, olives, and feta.
3. Stuff peppers, drizzle with olive oil and lemon juice.

Prep Time: *25 minutes*

✓ *Quinoa and black beans offer protein and fiber.*

✓ *Tomatoes and olives provide antioxidants.*

✓ *Feta adds a touch of calcium.*

Anti-Aging Spinach and Walnut Pesto Pasta:

Ingredients:

- Whole-grain or chickpea pasta
- Fresh spinach, walnuts, garlic
- Olive oil, nutritional yeast

Instructions:

1. Blend spinach, walnuts, garlic, olive oil, and nutritional yeast for pesto.
2. Cook pasta according to package instructions.
3. Toss pasta with pesto and serve.

Prep Time: *25 minutes*

✓ *Whole-grain or chickpea pasta offers fiber.*

✓ *Spinach provides vitamins and iron.*

✓ *Walnuts offer omega-3 fatty acids.*

Grilled Lemon Rosemary Salmon:

Ingredients:

- Salmon fillets
- Lemon, fresh rosemary
- Garlic, olive oil, salt, and pepper
- Quinoa or wild rice

Instructions:

1. Marinate salmon with lemon, rosemary, and garlic.
2. Grill until cooked, basting with olive oil.
3. Serve over quinoa or wild rice.

Prep Time: *30 minutes*

- ✓ *Salmon provides omega-3 fatty acids.*
- ✓ *Lemon and rosemary add flavor and antioxidants.*
- ✓ *Quinoa or wild rice offers complex carbs.*

Sweet Potato and Chickpea Curry:

Ingredients:

- ✓ *Sweet potatoes, chickpeas*

✓ *Coconut milk*

✓ *Onion, garlic, ginger*

✓ *Curry powder, turmeric, cumin*

✓ *Fresh cilantro, lime wedges*

Instructions:

1. Sauté onion, garlic, and ginger. Add sweet potatoes and chickpeas.
2. Stir in curry powder, turmeric, and cumin.
3. Serve over brown rice.

Prep Time: *35 minutes*

✓ *Chickpeas provide protein and fiber.*

✓ *Sweet potatoes offer vitamins and fiber.*

✓ *Turmeric and cumin have anti-inflammatory properties.*

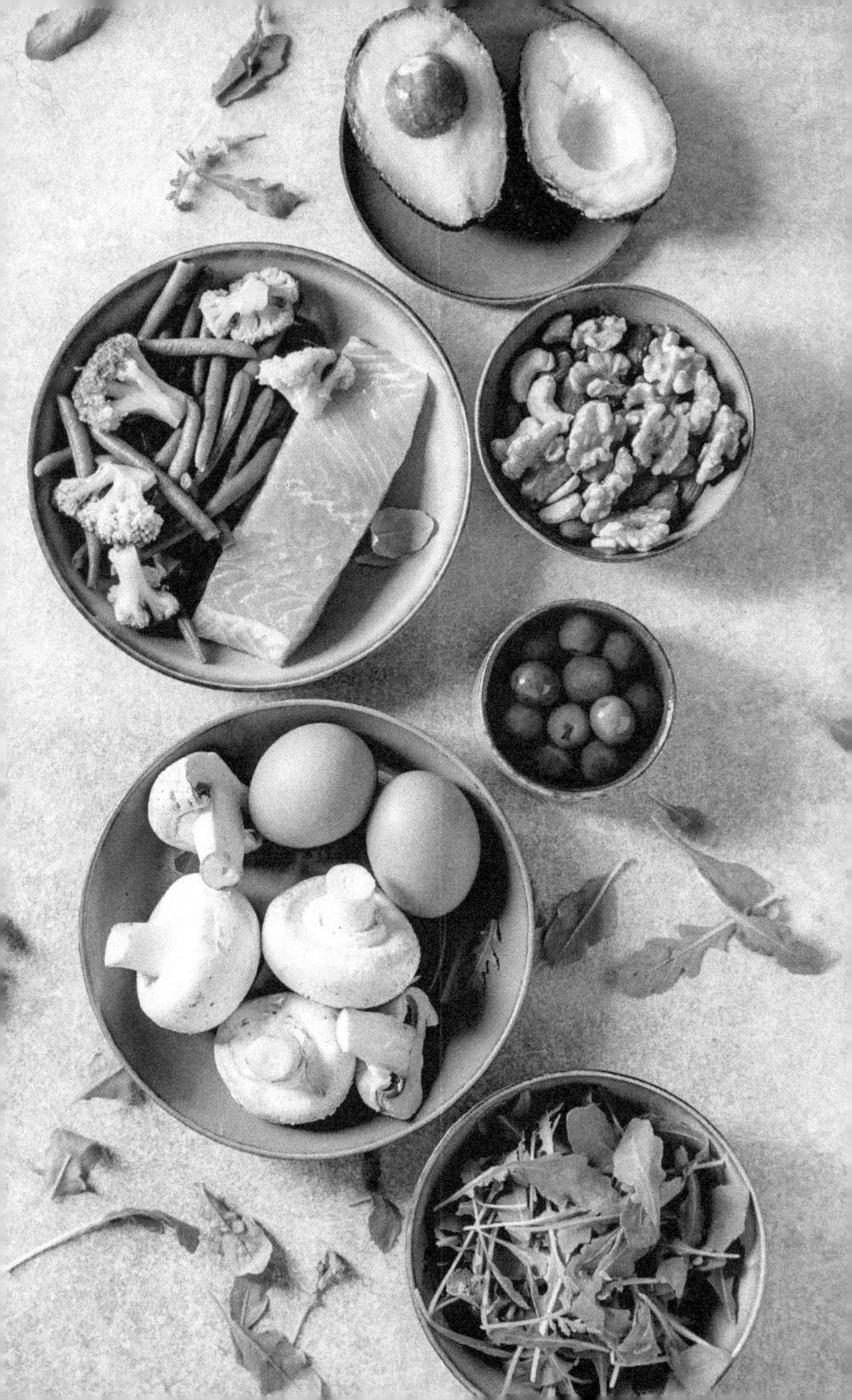

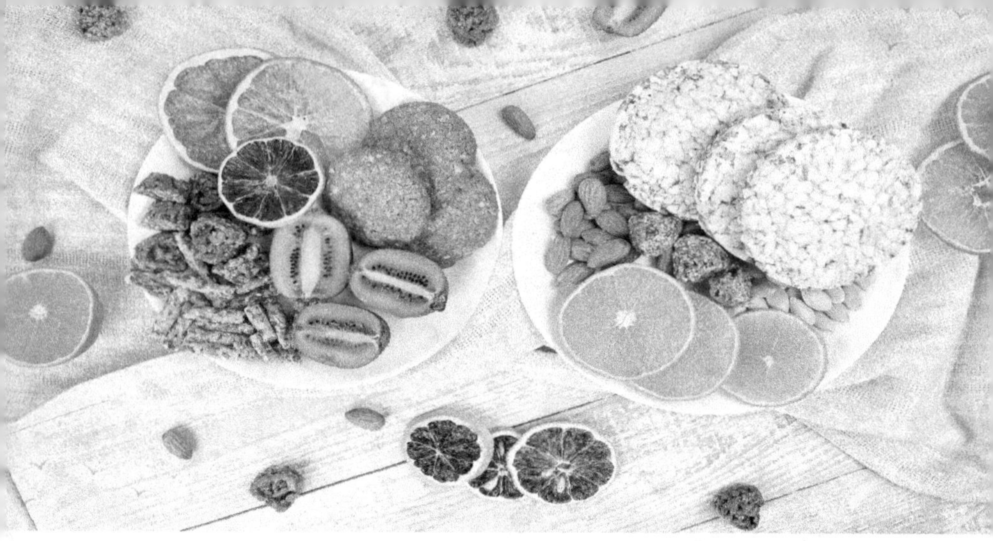

CHAPTER 5: SNACKS AND APPETIZERS WITH PURPOSE

Mediterranean Hummus Platter:

Ingredients:

- Hummus
- Cherry tomatoes, cucumber, bell peppers (sliced)
- Kalamata olives, feta cheese
- Whole-grain pita or crackers

Instructions:

1. Arrange hummus in the center of a platter.
2. Surround with sliced vegetables, olives, and feta.

3. Serve with whole-grain pita or crackers.

Prep Time: *15 minutes*

✓ *Hummus provides plant-based protein.*

✓ *Vegetables offer vitamins and fiber.*

✓ *Olive oil in hummus supports heart health.*

Plant-Powered Guacamole:

Ingredients:

- Avocado, tomatoes, red onion (diced)
- Cilantro, lime juice, garlic
- Whole-grain tortilla chips

Instructions:

1. Mash avocado, mix with tomatoes, red onion, and cilantro.
2. Add lime juice and minced garlic, stir well.
3. Serve with whole-grain tortilla chips.

Prep Time: *20 minutes*

✓ *Avocado provides healthy fats.*

✓ *Tomatoes offer antioxidants.*

✓ *Whole-grain chips add fiber.*

Turmeric Spiced Chickpea Roast:

Ingredients:

- Roasted chickpeas
- Turmeric, cumin, paprika, cayenne
- Olive oil, sea salt

Instructions:

1. Toss chickpeas with olive oil and spices.
2. Roast until crispy, sprinkle with sea salt.
3. Let cool and serve as a crunchy snack.

Prep Time: *25 minutes:*

✓ *Chickpeas provide protein and fiber.*

✓ *Turmeric has anti-inflammatory properties.*

✓ *Spices add flavor and health benefits.*

Mediterranean Stuffed Grape Leaves:

Ingredients:

- Grape leaves (canned or fresh)
- Quinoa, pine nuts, dried cranberries
- Lemon juice, olive oil, fresh dill

Instructions:

1. Mix cooked quinoa with pine nuts and dried cranberries.
2. Spoon the mixture onto grape leaves and roll.
3. Drizzle with lemon juice, olive oil, and garnish with dill.

Prep Time: *30 minutes*

- ✓ *Quinoa offers complete protein.*
- ✓ *Pine nuts provide healthy fats.*
- ✓ *Grape leaves offer antioxidants.*

Antioxidant-Packed Berry Bowl:

Ingredients:

- Mixed berries (blueberries, strawberries, raspberries)
- Greek yogurt or plant-based yogurt
- Chia seeds, honey or maple syrup

Instructions:

1. Arrange mixed berries in a bowl.
2. Top with a dollop of Greek or plant-based yogurt.
3. Sprinkle with chia seeds and drizzle with honey or maple syrup.

Prep Time: 15 minutes

- ✓ *Berries are rich in antioxidants.*
- ✓ *Greek yogurt provides protein.*
- ✓ *Chia seeds offer omega-3 fatty acids.*

Plant-Based Spinach and Artichoke Dip:

Ingredients:

- Fresh spinach, artichoke hearts (chopped)
- Cashews, nutritional yeast, garlic
- Lemon juice, almond milk

Instructions:

1. Blend cashews, nutritional yeast, garlic, and almond milk until smooth.
2. Sauté spinach and artichoke hearts, mix with the creamy blend.
3. Serve with vegetable sticks or whole-grain crackers.

Prep Time: *25 minutes*

- ✓ *Cashews provide plant-based protein.*
- ✓ *Spinach and artichokes offer vitamins.*
- ✓ *Nutritional yeast adds a cheesy flavor.*

Mediterranean Chickpea Bruschetta:

Ingredients:

- Toasted whole-grain baguette slices
- Cherry tomatoes, cucumber, red onion (diced)
- Chickpeas, olive oil, balsamic glaze

Instructions:

1. Mix diced vegetables with chickpeas and olive oil.
2. Spoon the mixture onto toasted baguette slices.
3. Drizzle with balsamic glaze before serving.

Prep Time: *20 minutes*

- ✓ *Chickpeas provide protein and fiber.*
- ✓ *Vegetables offer vitamins and antioxidants.*
- ✓ *Whole-grain baguette adds complex carbs.*

Golden Turmeric Edamame:

Ingredients:

- Edamame (steamed)
- Turmeric, garlic powder, sea salt

1. Toss steamed edamame with turmeric and garlic powder.
2. Sprinkle with sea salt and serve as a savory snack.

Prep Time: *10 minutes*

✓ *Edamame is rich in plant-based protein.*
✓ *Turmeric has anti-inflammatory properties.*
✓ *Sea salt adds flavor without excess sodium.*

Quinoa and Cucumber Sushi Rolls:

Ingredients:

- Nori sheets, cooked quinoa
- Cucumber, avocado, carrot (julienned)
- Soy sauce, wasabi, pickled ginger

1. Place quinoa and julienned vegetables on a nori sheet.
2. Roll tightly and slice into bite-sized pieces.
3. Serve with soy sauce, wasabi, and pickled ginger.

Prep Time: *30 minutes*

✓ *Quinoa provides complete protein.*

✓ *Vegetables offer vitamins and fiber.*

✓ *Nori sheets provide minerals.*

Stuffed Mini Bell Peppers:

Ingredients:

- Mini bell peppers (halved)
- Hummus or black bean dip
- Cherry tomatoes, fresh basil

Instructions:

1. Fill mini bell pepper halves with hummus or black bean dip.

2. Top with a cherry tomato and fresh basil leaf.

3. Arrange on a platter and serve.

Prep Time: *20 minutes*

✓ *Bell peppers offer vitamins and antioxidants.*

✓ *Hummus or black bean dip provides protein.*

✓ *Basil adds flavor and nutrients.*

Chia Seed Pudding Parfait:

Ingredients:

- Chia seed pudding (made with almond milk)
- Mixed berries, sliced kiwi
- Granola, coconut flakes

Instructions:

1. Layer chia seed pudding with mixed berries and sliced kiwi.

2. Sprinkle each layer with granola and coconut flakes.

3. Repeat layers and serve in a glass or bowl.

Prep Time: *15 minutes*

✓ *Chia seeds offer omega-3 fatty acids.*

✓ *Berries are rich in antioxidants.*

✓ *Almond milk provides plant-based calcium.*

Mediterranean Stuffed Mushrooms:

Ingredients:

- Button mushrooms (cleaned and stems removed)
- Quinoa, sun-dried tomatoes, black olives (chopped)
- Garlic, fresh parsley, olive oil

Instructions:

1. Mix quinoa with sun-dried tomatoes, black olives, garlic, and fresh parsley.
2. Spoon the mixture into each mushroom cap.
3. Drizzle with olive oil and bake until mushrooms are tender.

Prep Time: *25 minutes*

✓ *Quinoa provides complete protein.*

✓ *Sun-dried tomatoes and black olives offer antioxidants.*

✓ *Mushrooms are rich in vitamins and minerals.*

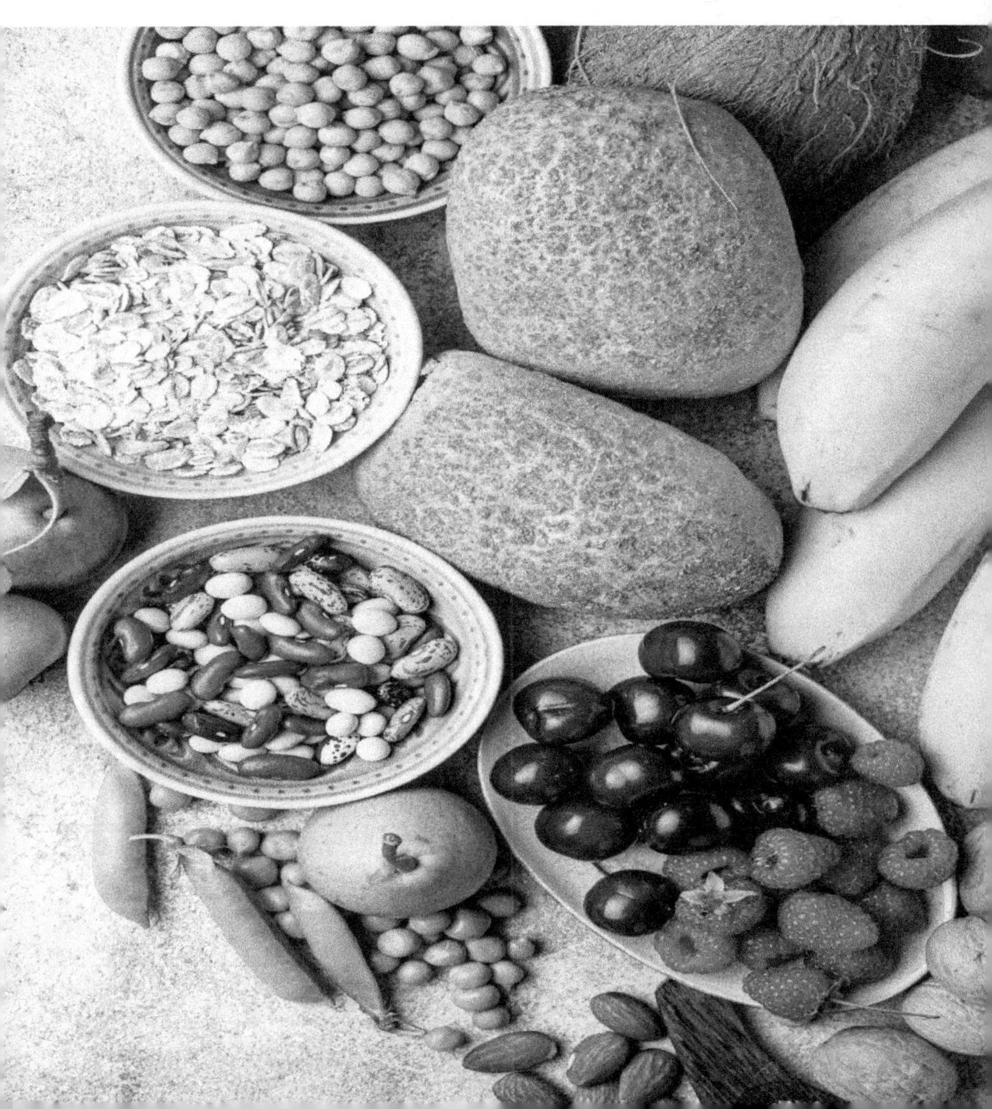

30-Day Meal Planning Challenge

Month

Meal Plan Schedule

DAY 1	DAY 2	DAY 3	DAY 4	DAY 5
DAY	DAY 7	DAY 8	DAY 9	DAY 10
DAY 11	DAY 12	DAY 13	DAY 14	DAY 15
DAY 16	DAY 17	DAY 18	DAY 19	DAY 20
DAY 21	DAY 22	DAY 23	DAY 24	DAY 25
DAY 26	DAY 27	DAY 28	DAY 29	DAY 30

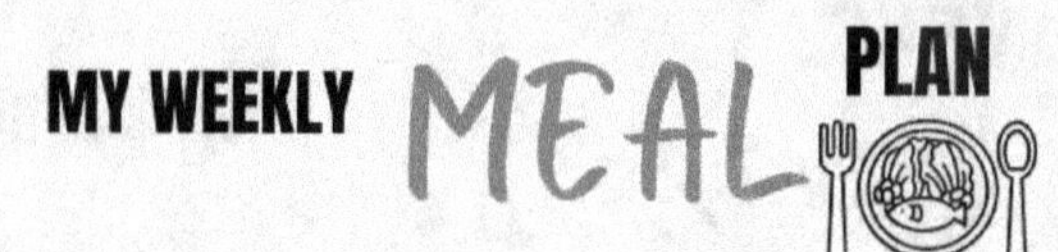

MEAL PLAN SCHEDULE

SNACKS

DRINKS

FRUITS

VEGETABLES

RECIPES

DATE: _______________

Recipe Name

- ☐ Mediterranean
- ☐ Plant-Based Diet
- ☐ Anti-Inflammatory
- ☐ Antioxidant-Rich

Prep Time

Cooking Time

Serve

Notes

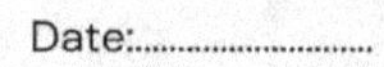

Personal *Journal*

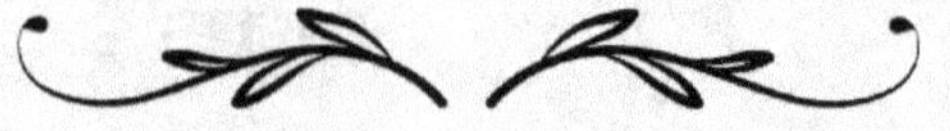

1	2	3	4	5	6
				MEETING	
7	8	9	10	11	12
13	14	15	16	17	18
19	20	21	22	23	24
25	26	27	28	29	30
		DON'T 4GET			

Note

Habit Tracker

Workout

Yoga

Eat Clean

Reflect on your personal beliefs and attitudes towards aging. How have these beliefs been shaped by societal norms, cultural influences, and personal experiences?

____

____

____

____

Imagine a world where aging is not a limiting factor. How would individuals approach their careers, relationships, and personal goals in such a society? Consider both the positive and potentially challenging aspects of this scenario.

____

____

____

____

Explore the concept of "aging gracefully." What does it mean to you, and how can individuals cultivate a positive and fulfilling life as they age, regardless of the number of years?

____

____

____

____

WEEK:

GROCERIES
LIST

....

....

....

....

....

....

....

....

....

....

....

....

MY WEEKLY MEAL PLAN

	BREAKFAST	LUNCH	DINNER
MONDAY			
TUESDAY			
WEDNESDAY			
THURSDAY			
FRIDAY			
SATURDAY			
SUNDAY			

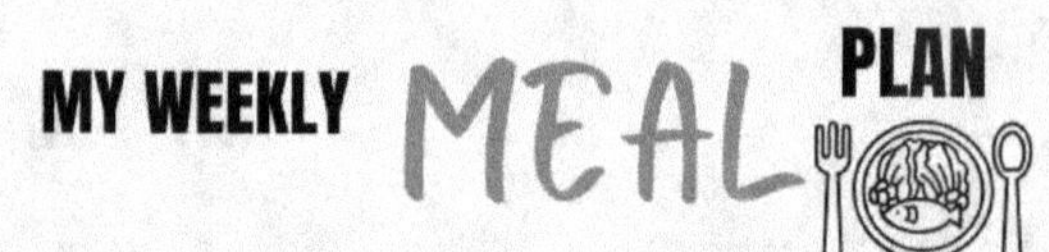

MEAL PLAN SCHEDULE

SNACKS

DRINKS

FRUITS

VEGETABLES

RECIPES

DATE: _______________

Recipe Name

☐ **Mediterranean**

☐ **Plant-Based Diet**

☐ **Anti-Inflammatory**

☐ **Antioxidant-Rich**

Prep Time

Cooking Time

Serve

Notes

....

....

....

....

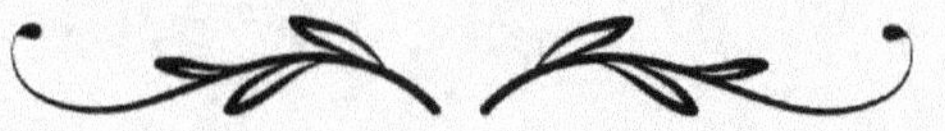

Personal *Journal*

1 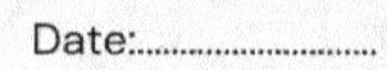	2	3	4	5 MEETING	6
7	8	9	10	11	12
13	14	15	16	17	18
19	20	21	22	23	24
25	26	27 DON'T 4GET	28	29	30

Note

....
....
....
....
....
....
....
....

Habit Tracker

Workout

Yoga

Eat Clean

Consider the role of mindfulness and stress management in promoting a healthier and potentially longer life. How can practices such as meditation and mindfulness positively impact the aging process?

____

____

____

____

Reflect on your own lifestyle choices, including diet, exercise, and sleep. How might adjusting these factors positively influence your overall well-being and potentially contribute to a longer, healthier life?

____

____

____

____

Imagine participating in a futuristic experiment aimed at slowing down the aging process. What ethical considerations would you take into account before deciding to undergo such an intervention? How might society respond to these interventions?

____

____

____

____

WEEK:

GROCERIES
LIST

MY WEEKLY MEAL PLAN

BREAKFAST	LUNCH	DINNER

MONDAY

TUESDAY

WEDNESDAY

THURSDAY

FRIDAY

SATURDAY

SUNDAY

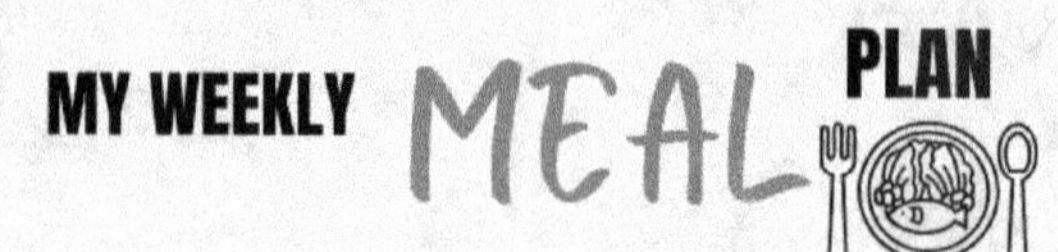

MEAL PLAN SCHEDULE

SNACKS

DRINKS

FRUITS

VEGETABLES

RECIPES

DATE: _______________

Recipe Name

- [ ] **Mediterranean**
- [ ] **Plant-Based Diet**
- [ ] **Anti-Inflammatory**
- [ ] **Antioxidant-Rich**

Prep Time

Cooking Time

Serve

Notes

Personal *Journal*

1	2	3	4	5	6
				MEETING	
7	8	9	10	11	12
13	14	15	16	17	18
19	20	21	22	23	24
25	26	27	28	29	30
		DON'T 4GET			

Note

....
....
....
....
....
....
....
....
....
....
....

Habit Tracker

Workout

Yoga

Eat Clean

Explore the idea of intergenerational relationships and their impact on well-being. How can connections with people of different ages contribute to a richer and more fulfilling life for individuals of all generations?

____

____

____

____

Consider the importance of purpose and meaning in life. How can having a sense of purpose influence the aging process, and what steps can individuals take to discover or cultivate meaning throughout their lives?

____

____

____

____

Reflect on the concept of a "midlife crisis." How might societal expectations and personal goals contribute to feelings of discontent in midlife, and what strategies can individuals employ to navigate this period positively?

____

____

____

____

WEEK:

GROCERIES LIST

BREAKFAST	LUNCH	DINNER	
			MONDAY
			TUESDAY
			WEDNESDAY
			THURSDAY
			FRIDAY
			SATURDAY
			SUNDAY

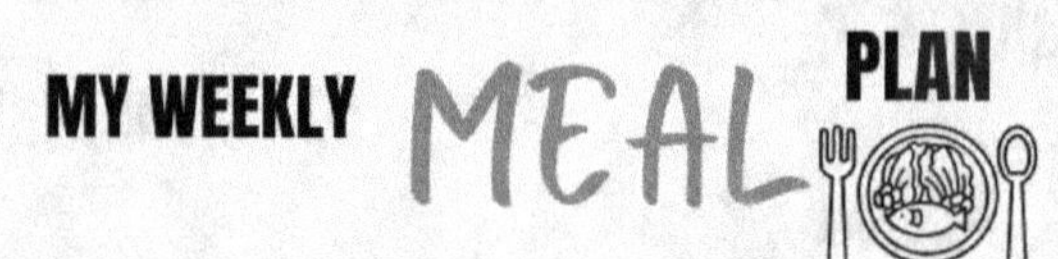

MEAL PLAN SCHEDULE

SNACKS

DRINKS

FRUITS

VEGETABLES

RECIPES

DATE: ______________

Recipe Name

- [ ] **Mediterranean**
- [ ] **Plant-Based Diet**
- [ ] **Anti-Inflammatory**
- [ ] **Antioxidant-Rich**

Prep Time

Cooking Time

Serve

Notes

....

....

....

....

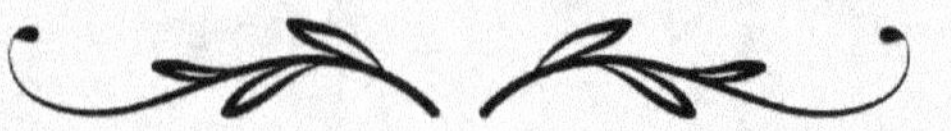

Personal *Journal*

Date:..........................

1	2	3	4	5 MEETING	6
7	8	9	10	11	12
13	14	15	16	17	18
19	20	21	22	23	24
25	26	27 DON'T 4GET	28	29	30

Note

Habit Tracker

Workout

Yoga

Eat Clean

Reflect on the concept of legacy and the mark individuals leave on the world. How can the pursuit of a meaningful legacy influence decisions and actions throughout one's life, particularly in the context of aging?

____

____

____

Explore the intersection of technology and aging. How can advancements in technology enhance the quality of life for older individuals? Consider potential innovations that could revolutionize healthcare, social connections, or daily living.

____

____

____

Investigate the impact of environmental factors on the aging process. How might the quality of the environment in which we live influence our health and longevity? Consider both physical and social aspects of the environment.

____

____

____

egetables

Legumes

Dairy
products

whole

grains

Seeds

Healthy

fats

CONCLUSION

Embracing a Lifespan Diet Lifestyle

Embracing a lifespan diet lifestyle is a transformative journey that transcends the conventional boundaries of nutrition. The "Lifespan Diet Cookbook" serves as a comprehensive guide, unraveling the intricacies of nutrition and its profound impact on our longevity. This lifestyle is not just about the food we consume; it is a holistic approach to nourishing both the body and mind, understanding that the choices we make today can shape the years ahead.

The role of nutrition in lifespan extension is elucidated throughout the cookbook, emphasizing the power of food as a key determinant of our overall well-being. From building a foundation of sustainable eating habits to delving into the intricacies of cellular health and its impact on longevity, the cookbook empowers readers to make informed choices that can potentially redefine their journey through the aging process.

Balancing macronutrients for optimal health becomes a guiding principle, showcasing that a harmonious blend of proteins, fats, and carbohydrates is the cornerstone of a resilient and vibrant life. The recipes provided, ranging from transformative breakfasts to wholesome lunches and delightful dinners, exemplify that longevity is not a distant goal but an achievable reality through mindful and purposeful eating.

Each recipe is crafted with intention, incorporating elements from the Mediterranean diet, plant-based philosophies, and the richness of anti-inflammatory and antioxidant-rich foods. These culinary creations not only tantalize the taste buds but also serve as a testament to the diversity and deliciousness that can be achieved within the realm of a lifespan diet.

By promoting a lifestyle that extends beyond mere sustenance, the cookbook invites individuals to become architects of their own health, architects who appreciate the profound connection between what is on their plate and the longevity of their existence. In this way, embracing a lifespan diet lifestyle becomes a celebration of the body's resilience, a commitment to the art of aging gracefully, and an acknowledgment that every meal is an opportunity to nurture not just the body, but the promise of a longer, healthier, and more fulfilling life. As we savor the flavors of these purposeful recipes, we embark on a journey towards a timeless and vibrant existence, understanding that the secret to a longer and more meaningful life may just be found in the very choices we make at the dinner table.

www.ingramcontent.com/pod-product-compliance
Lightning Source LLC
Chambersburg PA
CBHW070909260726
48661CB00004B/1677